Ylang Ylang &

Geranium

Essential oils

Trusting the Heart of Our Innocence

By: Stasia Bliss

This book may be shared in part or in its entirety by any means. You don't need permission from the author, for you and the author are ONE in the Divine Human Family. Use discretion and kindness.

3

This book and all the books in this series are dedicated to the ever renewed birthing of the Divine Self – for which the gifts of essential oils are continually given.

Table of Contents:

Caution - - Disclaimer - - Personal Health Observation -

This book is not a replacement for therapy, medicines, or treatments of any kind. It is merely meant to give a new perspective on the uses of the essential oil mentioned herein.

It is advised that through realizing yourself to be the only One you can change, that when things seem bleak or undesirable, when health or life seems to oppose you, that you instead choose to seek to affect change within yourself rather than look outward for "cures." This book in no way intends to heal or cure you or act as a replacement for medical or psychological treatment, it does intend to lift and inspire you into your own greatness and sovereignty. Proceed at your own risk and free-agency.

Introduction

"And the day came when the risk to remain tight in a bud

was more painful than the risk it took to blossom."

~ Anais Nin

Within these pages lies a challenge to the heart. You, the reader, will be asked to penetrate the often constructed barriers placed around the body's most tenderly brilliant organ and to urge it to open, trust and play again as it did when you were a child. This book will introduce you to your heart in a way you perhaps have never imagined and will show you how, through the simple application of essential oils, your heart can take you to the next level of experience, love and miracles.

That's right. Hold on to your ability to let go of the old and open up to seal in the wisdom that is hereto forthcoming.

Some call the heart the "second brain" but the truth is, it's the first one. As an embryo, your heart started beating before your brain started cognizing and it is still first in the steps you take to face challenges, overcome obstacles and embrace truths.

By understanding our most vital organ and the center point of our body's energy channels, we can tune into the life that is awaiting us, behind walls of regrets and fears, and beyond the shadows of yesterday's knowledge.

This book introduces you to two very special essential oils which love to work hand in hand on the heart and what it really has to teach us about love. This next book in the series of *Essential oils for Consciousness* takes us to the heart of the matter and to the heart itself, awaiting its potentiality behind walls of doubt and make believe grown-up ways.

Welcome to the journey of Ylang Ylang and Geranium.

Ylang Ylang and Geranium are both beautiful flowers, and with their help, the heart can learn to blossom, just as they do, to express authentically and love inclusively.

The Vibration and Power of the Heart

"Sometimes the heart sees what is invisible to the eyes."
~ H. Jackson Brown Jr.

The heart is an amazing organ. And beyond just the organ itself, the heart is a mechanism for human love and divine compassion, healing and manifestation. However, if the heart (and the energy center of the heart chakra) is blocked or inhibited in function, the entire body as well as surrounding entities can suffer.

An institution known as HeartMath has been studying the field emitted by the heart and has been able to measure it with high tech equipment to show how profoundly simple it is to affect change in the body and the atmosphere by focusing attention on the heart.

They have found that the heart emits a field which reaches about eight to ten feet around a person in every direction. This is confirmed by ancient teachings of the body sheaths in yogic philosophy, that the heart does in fact radiate a field of energy which overlaps and interacts with those who come near to us and live in our environment.

You know when you go into a room that you can feel the energy in that room almost immediately. This is because you are able to tap into the energy in the room and the prevalent energy of every person's heart vibration through the sensitivity of your own heart field. The heart-field is made to read, download and give feedback into your personal awareness regarding the other energies prevalent in the area and signal to you whether such interaction is "desirable" or not.

We know when we are in a place that feels good and that seems to resonate with our own being completely. There is nothing nicer than finding yourself in a coherent field of positive intent. When many like-minded and like-hearted people gather together, their collective fields affect the environment in so much as they create a field of common intent, amplified by the loving vibrations felt in their hearts.

The HeartMath Institute has found that when a person holds feelings of love, gratitude, appreciation and praise in the heart, their heart waves and brain waves move into a coherent state. This coherence affects the entire body in a healthy, positive way and helps to contribute to wellness and longevity. When a group of people are in coherence, it has been found that it takes no more than .01% of a population to affect positive change through combining positive fields of intent through the heart.

The Maharishi Effect is the name given to the effects generated by a group meditating together with intentions and feelings of peace. Originally discovered by groups of Transcendental Meditation practitioners, these groups have had such a profound effect on their environment and surrounding cities that crime rates reportedly dropped significantly and emergency room visits went down during the time of peace held in the hearts of a small group at once.

In yogic philosophy, the heart chakra is said to be the center in the physical body responsible for unconditional love, compassion, healing and even wish-fulfillment. Sages of old have reported that when an individual is in alignment with the higher will of life, a "greater power," or "Source," and has risen above the tendencies of the "lower centers" – or those having to do with self-desires, base instincts and negative patterning; one's very wishes could be fulfilled because of the field into which they have tapped.

The heart is being realized to be a powerful organ indeed. Researchers, doctors, teachers and individuals alike are starting to recognize the innate wisdom and healing potential which lies in the heart of every man, woman and child. It is no mistake that our hearts develop first, as the key to both our awareness and our physical existence. The heart must be felt, purely, deeply, and unencumbered by the falsities that we may use to cloak this powerful center throughout our lives.

Often, we find ourselves in life, afraid of being hurt emotionally. Our vulnerability leaves us at the mercy of other's actions and freedom to reject the very love we seek to give. When we experience heartache multiple times, we may unconsciously block the heart from emitting its powerful waves of intent and instead send out a very different vibration.

It takes some wisdom (and sometimes negative experiences), to realize how important it is to live with a heart free and unblocked by negative emotions and patternings. Most of us have taken on a block or two over the years, finding it crucial, at times, to protect our vulnerable and deep expanse of love.

Now is the time we must realize the power lying buried in the heart and awaken the child within, who has hidden for fear of falling. We must learn to trust life and others again so we may experience reality from a place of awe and wonderment like we did as children. No matter the happenings we have faced and felt, no matter the hardships and rejections, the power which can be found in an open heart is worth uncovering. The child within awaits the chance to run free and show us that life is full of joy and can be trusted, it must be trusted... for without trust, no magic may be discovered.

Let us explore the common heart wall protection so many of us resort to, what it is made of and how we may bring it down gracefully.

Heart-wall Protection

From the first time you were ever told not to feel what you were feeling, whether verbally or energetically, until now... slowly and gradually a wall was constructed around your precious and powerful heart. Not only that, the sweet, innocent child-self aspect of you who knew how to connect to Source energy, trusted life and spontaneously valued play... that inner child was removed from her rightful place in your heart and took a seat slightly outside of you, above your physical, and was thoughtfully renamed "your higher self."

Meanwhile, the heart has been beating on the inner walls of your being, asking to be heard, sending signals of heart throbs toward certain dreams and aspirations. Something, anything, to get your attention so you would find a way to deconstruct this wall built around your heart.

Now, it was no mistake that your heart was protected the way it has been. Nothing is a mistake in the journey of evolution and awakening. However, the time is now to take down the barriers surrounding your heart and allow pure divine love to both be given and received by you. It is what you were meant for.

Over time, unprocessed emotions which felt potentially injurious to our hearts were used as fortress walls to prevent any further damage to our tender and loving hearts. All it took was one unpleasant experience and one painful heartache for our psyche to decided we needed back-up. Our hearts would no longer be subject to the untrustworthy emotions of others and instead we would be safe behind walls of previous emotions we did not care to integrate. True?

Well, one thing is certain; each and every one of us has had a wall constructed around our hearts. These walls have been built of trapped emotions and have protected us from hurt, but they have also protected us from greater love.

The time has come to learn to trust again and to let that inner child run free once more. This is possible by releasing stuck emotions around the heart, lowering the walls and bringing in the vibrations which would support trust and authenticity, like those frequencies found by using ylang ylang and geranium essential oils.

Geranium and Trust

Geranium

This lump in my throat Jumps. Almost as if it wants

To say something.

I did not know what it is.

I feel I need to measure some sort of emotion, but what it is...

And it scares me.

I feel the vultures and crow

Just waiting for the right moment.

I should feel warm, I am alive right?

Because you can see me, can't you?

You are my Geranium.

-The New Kestral

Geranium essential oil has the power to instill new trust in both ourselves and our ability to love, but also in those who would come into our fields.

As we drop the emotions which block our tender hearts, geranium becomes a powerful tool to use in building strength in the heart and opening doorways of potential so our hearts may learn to feel and love again.

It takes a great deal of trust to open the vulnerabilities of the heart after it has been closed down and blocked. If not properly cared for, even if the heart is opened with other modalities, it could close again if it feels it unsafe. The heart must learn to trust in life and love and the process of feeling again. This trust is only earned through experiences planted in the soil of good faith and strong vibrations.

Geranium essential oil is rich in floral notes and is akin to giving yourself bouquets of flowers en masse. At first it can be overwhelming to receive so much. The vibration is high and the depth of wealth in just a few drops, in even one drop of geranium, is sometimes more than a person can seem to take in.

At first, it may be necessary to dilute geranium a lot. To put it in a bottle of almond oil or coconut oil and allow the fragrance to be diffused a bit. Trust cannot be built up all in one day or in one dose. It is a gradual process of slowly feeding the fragrance into your field. It is a romance between your heart and the world again and geranium is the balm that guards against potential hurts re-injuring.

Keeping geranium, in diluted form, on wrist points and over the high heart can help to increase the potential for trust to be experienced in the world with those who come into your field and into the environment. The tendency will be to remain open, after using geranium for a time, where you might have closed off sooner before.

Geranium inspires a sense of emotional maturity. It raises the bar for those things which you can handle. Perhaps it is the pungency of its scent that allows for this. It seems to take a mature nose to take in and "handle" its fragrance for long or often. By the same token, this oil is demanding of our emotional nature, to raise the bar and allow for more growth and flexibility.

Geranium inspires greatness and it does so by giving the sense of accomplishment for being able to make room to trust again. Trusting comes from vulnerability, but the trust inspired by geranium is not naïve in being vulnerable, it is a smart, savvy trust that comes from a higher awareness. One who gains trust with geranium essential oil has gained the insight of a higher vision. The trust comes from trusting life and the benevolence of a higher power, not the personalities that run around in disguise as humans with names.

As geranium essential oil is used, life will naturally feel like a kinder place as curiosity replaces negative emotional reactions. Even if a situation proves to be unworthy of your love or affection, disappointment will only be for the needed change yet again, but trust will not be shattered, for trust will have been built for the ultimate reality, which cannot so easily be shattered by simple human mistakes and the mishaps of love.

As trust is reinstilled into a person, geranium will not be needed as often, but may also be used, when chosen, in a less diluted form.

Geranium essential oil connects the heart chakra to the first and earth chakras – helping to ground love in a very real and tangible way. The heart and high heart are supported by this oil and any heart-walls that may have been constructed are urged to weaken and be understood and released.

Ylang Ylang & Accepting the Child Within

The sweet smell of ylang ylang essential oil is reminiscent of childhood, running through wildflowers and stringing them through your hair. This precious oil holds innocence and laughter, freedom and authenticity as its secret gift.

As the heart learns to trust life again, it is once more admitted through the sacred corridors of bliss and spontaneity that are so long associated with childhood and youthful wonder. The restless inner child whom we have inadvertently set aside in favor of a more "mature" and "grounded" reality wrought with logic and linearity is patiently awaiting our admission of error for leaving her behind.

It isn't that our grown-up world does not have some credence and need for us to place our feet firmly upon the ground as opposed to upside-down on the tire swing, it is just that we cannot live on the timeline of no imagination all the time. We are creative beings, divine beings and have an almost desperate need within our bodies to acknowledge and play with the child-self somehow in our waking lives.

Sure, nobody expects us to live completely from our child-self, and if we did, there would likely be just as big of a problem as we are in without this delightful aspect of us in balanced expression, but note the key word here – balance.

While carefully constructing protective devises around our precious hearts the child within was rather rudely retired to the look-out tower of impracticality. Rather than playing in harmony with the rest of the inner family – complete with the inner nurturer, the inner warrior and the inner sage – the inner child has felt to be off in the corner somewhere only consulted as an after-thought of "higher promptings" when otherwise uncertain.

Ylang ylang essential oil helps us to reconnect with the heart of childhood. That part of us that trusted in the benevolence of life and tuned into magic and imagination.

The most beautiful part about utilizing ylang ylang essential oil is that it helps to reignite the innocence of childhood discovery for those things you love in your life now. It becomes as though you are seeing them fresh again, with the enthusiasm of youth and the appreciation of the untarnished heart.

When used in meditation or in the presence of others, ylang ylang essential oil helps to open up the vital lines of communication – either to the Divine, Inner-child, "higher" self, or to the person or people we are with.

As the energies around the heart are cleared and trust begins to take root in your being again by using geranium essential oil, ylang ylang plays a harmonious role in inviting vigor and spontaneity to the mature wisdom that geranium offers. Trust in life is felt from almost opposing angles, and a person is genuinely brought into a sense of peace with life and the emotions allowed to be experienced with a body.

With the help of geranium and ylang ylang essential oils, love can more beautifully and simply take root in your life and those feelings that might block the path of the evolution of love and connectivity will suddenly be dispersed, replaced by the curiosity of possibility.

Ylang ylang can also be used in diluted form to start, as well as diffused into the environment in order to inspire playful imagination, and a connection to the youthful viewpoint of surrender and awe.

Trusting Joy Again

As a child, few of us had issues trusting joy or deciding to play and use our imaginations. As we grew and took on patterns and emotions impressed upon us which, over time, began to weigh us down, there became less and less possibility for us to trust life and trust joy. As the burdens grew, life started to feel all too serious and the pathway to joy, more cluttered and less accessible.

The amazing thing about essential oils is that they raise the vibration of the field of your body. They uplift the frequency you live in. No matter where you are experiencing life from before the use of essential oils, you will – without a doubt – shift your reality exponentially through the use of oils to one that is healthier and more joyful than you ever imagined possible.

We all live within fields of energy. Our bodies are made up of energy. We are molecules, dancing with vibration.

Depending on the other "factors" of our environment, including the foods we eat, the thoughts we have and the other input we give ourselves (or are exposed to) the sum total of these inputs will determine our health and our joy quotient.

Essential oils affect your energy field. They raise the vibration so significantly that they can even help to cancel out some of the negative patterning in the environment. Essential oils like geranium and ylang ylang help to bring in a vibration which can literally flip your reality from one you may not desire to one you do – in a fairly short amount of time – when used regularly.

By simply diffusing these beautifully fragrant oils into your environment you are, in effect, inviting the innocence of the child-self back into your life and intending on joy to become a more constant companion.

When in the presence of these sweet oils, one cannot help but feel uplifted and inspired, creative and full of life. Geranium instills trust and Ylang ylang reconnects one with the playful nature of youth. Together, they are the yin and yang of flower oils. Both pungent and sweet, together they make the heart available for love again and ready to dance in the field of opportunity where before only walls and fences lived.

Best Applications

Topically –

If you have sensitive skin you can dilute in coconut oil or other base oil. You need only a drop or two of these gorgeous floral oils. A little can go a very long, long way. Rub over areas of tension or constriction, especially heart, wrists and neck points. Imagine the heart opening and vibrancy coming forth.

Breathe it in –

Diffusing these precious oils into the atmosphere can help the blocks around the heart to begin to dissolve, inviting a new experience of trust and calmness into the scene. The scent is an invitation to step with trust into love and connection and it is recommended to use in rooms where intimacy would occur.

Geranium oil might be diffused into an environment where you would sit with a date or loved one you are seeking to cultivate trust with. Ylang ylang is great in kids rooms or in common areas of a house to foster healthy play and interaction.

Over the heart and high heart Chakras –

To assist in the activation and purification of the heart and high heart chakras/energy centers you can apply these oils right to the sternum and collar bone region. Dilute in a base oil first and then dab a tiny bit of either one or both oils mixed to this area. When doing so, imagine opening up the heart and high heart to express more purely from a place of trust and innocent knowing.

Souls of the Feet – applied to the feet, these oils can assist one in interacting spontaneously and tall upon the Earth and feeling the supportive energies available to all from the core of the great Mama. If one is feeling stuck, unable to move due to a lack of trust in life, geranium applied to the soles of the feet can help one get unstuck and move with greater fluidity. If there is a heaviness to walking and a tendency to feel "old" or in a rut, Ylang ylang applied to the feet can inspire a lightness to the step and playfulness in mood and expression.

Top of the Head, third eye and temples –

Applied to the head in these various spots, these flower oils can inspire mental and spiritual connection to the truth of childlike expression and surrendered trust. A greater vision within can be opened so one might begin to envision a world where individuals are connected to their ability to trust and play and a pathway might be created to this vision, coming through the one envisioning.

Third-eye empowerment is especially powerful with these oils as they help one to embody the child-self as well as the mature partner all at once both within the heart – through the scent, and through the higher mind of awareness through this vital center – directly connected to the pineal gland.

Divine Child of the Universe, anoint thyself with oils for thine own remembrance, for Ye are Gods!

Geranium for the Body:

Tones the skin

Tightens the gums

Helps fight cold sores

Contracts blood vessels

Antibacterial and antimicrobial

Facilitates blood flow under the skin's surface

Tightens pores

Helps to fade scars

Melanin- uniform distribution of

Wound healer

Astringent

Stop Hemorrhaging

Ylang ylang for the Body:

Antiseptic

Antidepressant

Lower blood pressure

Sedative – relief from stress and anxiety, insomnia

Nervine –soothes and protects nervous system

Helps balance blood pressure

Aphrodisiac

Colic

Heart arrhythmia

Hormonal Balance

Diabetes support – over pancreas

Hair loss

Resources:

Maharishi Effect: MUM ~ Maharishi University of Management

(www.mum.edu)

HeartMath.org – fields around heart

Global Coherence Initiative – Heart fields

Inner family – Alminewisdom.com

doTERRA essential oils – www.doterrauniversity.com

To buy oils visit –www.mydoterra.com/blissinthehouse

My personal website: www.blissinthehouse.com

www.ingramcontent.com/pod-product-compliance
Lightning Source LLC
Chambersburg PA
CBHW070508290526
45790CB00003B/1148